Paleo Diet – Don't Harm Yourself

How to Avoid TOP 5 Mistakes on the Paleo Diet, Paleo Guide for Beginners, Meal Plan for Weight Loss, 30 Tasty Recipes, Paleo Lifestyle, and Body Healing

WAIT...

Before You Continue, Here Is The Deal! If You Read It To The End Of The Book I Will Give Away A Bonus Of 4 Valuable Reports For Weight Loss and Healthy Eating (Value $27) FOR FREE!

Actually, I want You to be more prepared for Paleo lifestyle, that's why I've decided to provide you a valuable free bonus as a reward for reading this book to the end. Also, in this way I want to thank you for choosing my book amongst all other books, so simply enjoy reading and this is what you will get as a reward:

- FEEL MORE FULL EATING LESS REPORT
- HEALTHY COOKING TIPS FOR BETTER WEIGHT LOSS REPORT
- LENTILS REPORT
- SODIUM AND HEALTH REPORT

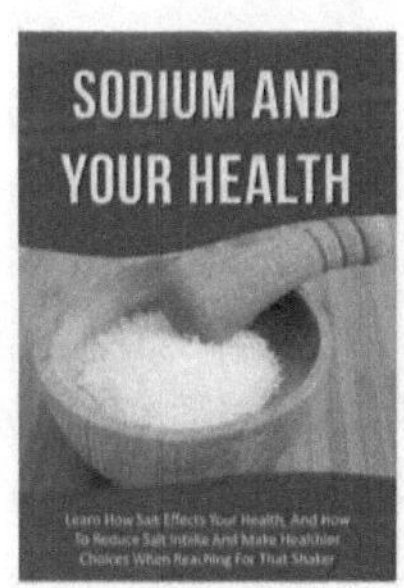

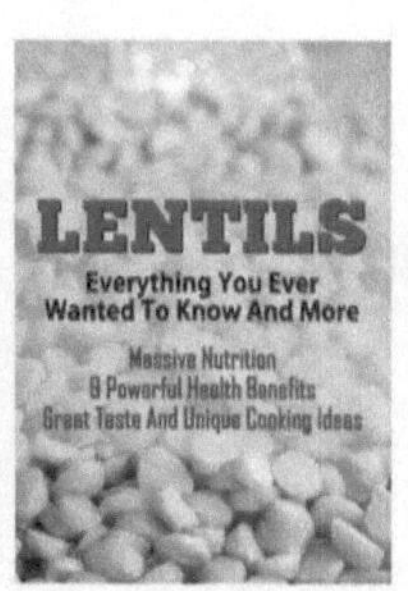

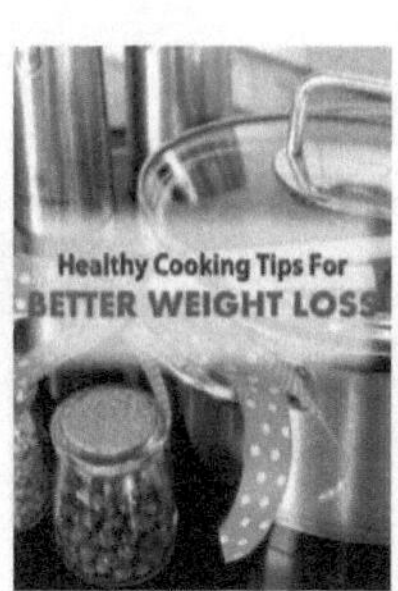

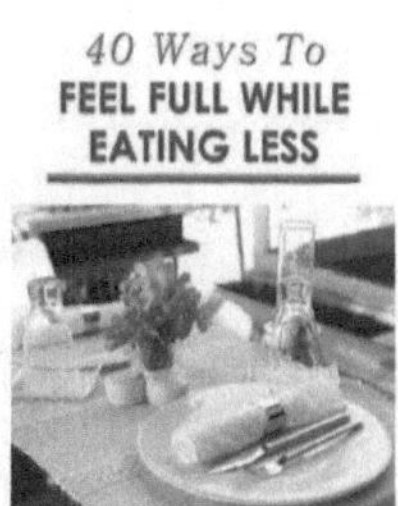

INSTRUCTIONS TO DOWNLOAD FREE REPORTS ARE IN THE END OF THE BOOK

Table of Contents

Introduction

Congratulations on getting a copy of *Paleo Diet – Don't Harm Yourself.* Thank you for doing so!

The following chapters will bring to light one of the most popular and renowned diets on the market today. The Paleo Diet is unlike all other diets in that it works alongside your genetics to boost your energy levels as well as assist you in achieving that strong, lean appearance almost everyone yearns for these days.

You will discover how important each part of the Paleo diet is as you venture throughout the upcoming chapters. You will find that this diet particularly leaves an exuberant amount of room for personalization. This is vital for those that already have a busy life and feel unmotivated to incorporate lots of rules in order to follow a diet. The Paleo diet is all about taking a step back in time to nourish ourselves in the ways our ancestors did. The cavemen did not have processed foods and easy to eat goodies. They worked hard to retrieve the food they could devour, and the Paleo is a direct representation of this past life.

The entirety of this book is written to be geared towards folks that wish to try out the Paleo diet and to quickly gather the must-do's and don'ts when it comes to implementing its methods into everyday life.

Along with lots of valuable information, there are delicious, easy to make recipes as well as a beginner's meal guide to get you started on the right foot as you begin your journey back in time, eating at the dinner table with our not-so-different cavemen ancestors!

There are plenty of books about the Paleo Diet on the market, so thanks again for choosing this one! Every effort was made to ensure it is full of as much useful information as possible. Please enjoy!

Chapter 1: The Basics of the Paleo Diet

If one is to simply Google "The Paleo Diet", a plethora of websites would eagerly fill up your search results, but many sites contain a bunch of things that are not 100% accurate, not true in the slightest, or are so complicated to read that it is an immediate turnoff from anyone wanting to try the diet out. I am here to tell you that the Paleo diet is actually quite simple and is easy to understand.

Simply put, anything that our caveman ancestors did not consume should be crossed off your list of acceptable consumables. So, I will inform you right now that if you are not quite ready to part with candy, cereal, pasta, and other similar foods, the Paleo diet is not for you...yet. The Paleo diet is based around foods that we as humans could either gather or hunt for. This means seeds, vegetables, leafy greens, nuts, fish, and meats are totally acceptable!

Within this chapter you will find the main guidelines you must follow in order to properly and successfully kick-start your way into the Paleolithic diet. While it is not totally for the weak at heart, if you are serious about losing weight and getting into possibly the best shape of your life, this diet is a tried and true one that if followed, can lead to great success in your physical life! Are you ready to really invest in your overall well-being and long-term health?

Paleo Diet Guidelines

High in fat but low in carbohydrates

To get the nutrients you need, you will also need to consume moderate levels of animal proteins as well. Luckily for you, one of the best features of the Paleo diet is that counting carbs and utilizing portion control is not necessary and is actually discouraged!

Be generous with saturated fats

Butter is encouraged on the Paleo! Other great (and healthier) options are coconut oil, beef or lamb tallow, lard, duck fat. Olive, macadamia, and avocado oils are also encouraged but should be utilized for drizzling and salads, not to cook with.

Consume lots of animal proteins

The Paleo diet is certainly not one that will leave you feeling light-headed. You are allowed to eat red meat, pork, eggs, poultry, animal organs, wild caught fish, and shellfish. Do not be hesitant when eating a fatty cut of meat. A great skill you may want to learn is to cook with bones in forms of broths and stocks.

Eat lots of fresh/frozen fruits veggies

Veggies are highly encouraged as part of the Paleo regimen. They can be fresh or frozen and can be either raw or cooked. You also do not have to worry about avoiding starchy veggies, since these are a good source of non-toxic carbs.

Consume small to moderate amounts of nuts and fruits

Ensure you consume fruits that are low in sugar but high in antioxidants. This is why berries and nuts are so popular on the Paleo diet, for they are high in omega-3's and low in omega-6's. If you want to lose weight at a faster rate, I suggest cutting out the majority of fruits altogether for quicker results.

Choose local meat

When picking meat to consume, lean towards grass-fed and pasture-raised options that come directly from environmentally conscious and local farms. The leaner the cut of meat, the better it is for you. You can supplement fat in the form of butter or coconut oil.

Avoid legumes and grains

I know, this one seems way easier said than done. But the caveman didn't have pre-made pasta, cereals, or any of these luxury foods that are actually trashing our bodies. Avoid all of these and anything similar:

- Black-eyes peas
- Navy beans
- Pinto beans
- Kidney beans
- Peanuts
- Soy
- Brown rice
- Corn
- Oats
- Barley
- Wheat
- Rye

Avoid hydrogenated and vegetable oils

- Sunflower oil
- Safflower oil
- Canola oil
- Peanut oil
- Corn oil
- Soybean oil
- Margarine

Yup, you got to avoid all of the above. Avocado and olive oil are still okay to consume, but make sure you use them to drizzle over food or as a component in salad dressing. Do not cook with them.

Cut out all sources of added sugar

This is another difficult task for many of us these days. We are all about convenience, and in those options, lies many added sugars and other additives. To truthfully conduct yourself on the Paleo, you must avoid all juices, packaged/processed sweets, soft drinks, and anything else that includes added sugar(s). I suggest that you visit the produce, fish, and meat sections for your main grocery shopping to avoid temptations.

Avoid dairy products

While heavy cream and butter are still a go on the Paleo, you will need to eliminate all other sources of dairy in your diet. If you are having a difficult time separating yourself from these items, there are fermented, full-fat, or raw options you can consider. But remember, the cavemen lived without these products, which means you can too!

Eat only when hungry

If you accidentally skip a meal or two, don't sweat. We have been programmed to think that we need three square meals each and every day. This is far from true. The cavemen spent days without eating as they hunted and gathered their next meal. Do what feels natural to you and stop forcing yourself to eat, even when you are not hungry.

Eliminate stressors

While easier said than done, erasing daily sources of stress from your life will lead you to make better choices, including what you put into your body. Strive for 8 hours of sleep each night and make it a habit to not sleep in past the chiming of your alarm clock in the morning.

Do not overdo exercise

In order to lose the most weight, it's important to remember that our bodies burn more fat by having short, intense workouts. Keep sessions short and perform them only a few times per week. If you do feel tired, don't overdo it. Learn to do short but intense sprinting sessions rather than long cardio.

How the Paleo Diet Works

Now that you know a few guidelines for success on the Paleo diet, you are probably wondering how in the world it actually works. The most popular reason people turn to the Paleo diet in order to lose weight is that it actually has the power to turn your body into a fat-burning machine rather than a carb-burning machine. The human body prefers to burn fat as its primary source of energy. This is because it burns slower and is more efficient for the body to utilize. But in today's world, the majority of our society consumes high amounts of carbohydrates rather than fat. When we intake more carbs than we need, our bodies turn it into fat and then store it for later use. Since our society is so advanced, we almost never have to face "not eating", which means our bodies do not necessarily know *how* to use up fat for fuel.

That being said, the Paleo diet does this pretty cool thing of rewiring our body's fuel system. By removing carbs from the diet, it can no longer get away with utilizing carbs for a source of energy, meaning it must use our excess fat for fuel. Isn't that awesome?! With the levels of carbs decreasing, your body's blood sugar balances out and regulates levels of insulin. With this action, the process of lipolysis happens. This means that our bodies release our triglycerides, or storage of fat, to be used as energy. So simply put, fewer carbs equals more fat being used up!

Acceptable Foods to Consume

- **Meat** – beef, lamb, chicken, turkey, pork, etc.
- **Fish and seafood** – shellfish, shrimp, haddock, trout, salmon
- **Eggs**
- **Vegetables** – tomatoes, carrots, onions, peppers, kale, broccoli, etc.
- **Fruits** – avocados, blueberries, strawberries, pears, oranges, bananas, apples, etc.
- **Tubers** – turnips, yams, sweet potatoes, potatoes, etc.
- **Nuts** – pumpkin, hazelnuts, walnuts, macadamia, almonds, etc.
- **Natural oils and healthy fats** – avocado oil, coconut oil, extra-virgin olive oil, etc.
- **Natural sweeteners** – honey, maple syrup, etc.
- **Salt and spices** – rosemary, turmeric, garlic, Himalayan salt, sea salt, etc.

Non-Acceptable Foods to Consume

- Vegetable oils
- Grains
- Dairy
- Legumes
- Refined carbohydrates
- Refined sugar
- Processed foods

Sensible Indulgences

- **Dark chocolate** – aim for chocolate with a 70% or higher in cocoa. Dark chocolate that is quality is healthy and nutritious!

- **Wine** – red wine is made up of healthy nutrients and antioxidants

When Thirsty

- **Tea** – Loaded with antioxidants, tea is very healthy. Aim to drink green tea as much as possible.

- **Coffee** – Also high in antioxidants, it has many good health benefits.

Chapter 2: How Anyone Can Begin the Paleo Diet

As we all know, it can be a real pain in the butt starting anything new. In regards to food especially, it can be a challenge to give up snacks and other goodies that make our taste buds feel good. You are probably overwhelmed by having to cut back on everyday choices and rewire your mindset to make healthier habits. Well, give yourself a pat on the back already, because you just got the first step out of the way. You have purchased this book in an effort to pave the way to a healthy lifestyle and you have now become acquainted with the basics of the Paleo diet!

Almost similar to an addict weaning off their addictive habits, you must take baby steps towards your goal in order to successfully stay the course. If you do not do this, you will probably end up going back to your old ways of late night snacking, binge-eating, and any other bad eating habits. So, this chapter is essentially for those of you that feel mighty overwhelmed in starting this whole Paleo diet journey. These steps will hopefully assist you in making the transition a bit easier on your mind and body.

Remove any irritating foods from your diet

This step will occur over the course of you performing the following steps as well. Focus on one thing at a time, such as gluten. This means cutting out and avoiding all foods that are under whatever category you are working on. If you decide to cut out gluten first, this means removing barley, oats, wheat, etc. Once you have successfully tackled one area, move on to the next, such as grains.

Get in the habit of cooking *all* your own meals

Out in the public world, it's quite difficult to find places to eat out at that will go consistently with your dieting principles. This is one of the most challenging aspects of any diet really, but especially the Paleo, since we are so used to convenience foods. Collect recipes that look good to you to prepare. I suggest making recipes that will result in large quantities so that you can have leftovers for throughout the week. If you really are ambitious, pick a day that you can prep and prepare all your meals throughout the week and freeze them. It is more convenient this way, as well as a major time/money saver.

Get used to the fact almost every meal will have protein and veggies

While fruits and nuts are allowed on the Paleo diet, really strive to incorporate protein and vegetables into almost every meal. Think of it as an opportunity to try out new things you otherwise would have never thought to consume.

Be conscious of carbs and added sugars

Once you have successfully cut out dairy, grains, and legumes from your diet, it's time to start looking into methods of reducing your carb intake. What other starches and sugars are still hiding amongst your diet? While starchy veggies are encouraged, you will need to greatly decrease any additional sugars.

Be conscious about fats

As you get more familiar with the Paleo diet, learn to cook with bacon fat, lard, tallow, or coconut oil and only use avocado, macadamia, and olive oils as a source of raw fat. Your consumption of omega-3's and omega-6's should be considered as well. If you are consuming lots of conventional meat, you may need to think about taking a fish oil supplement.

Look at quality of food

By cutting out pre-packed, convenient, and sugary foods, you already did yourself a huge favor. But if there are still processed food chemicals in your diet, like deli meats and bacon, it is time to remove these too. A big part of being successful on the Paleo diet is thinking about where your food actually comes from. If your budget allows, strive for grass-fed, organic, wild-caught fish, pasteurized eggs, locally grown and fruits/vegetables that are currently in season.

Purge the pantry

As you go through all the above steps, make sure you are throwing out all the foods you are no longer consuming to avoid future temptation. In fact, a better way to get rid of all that food is to donate to a local food bank.

Find and utilize support

A lack of understanding from family and friends is one of the biggest factors that keep people from sticking to diets and/or creating healthier habits for themselves. Search for resources online where you can post/add questions and comments or find some people that are in the same boat as you! Feeling as if you are a member of a community will help you to cope with changes and will also give you a sense of accountability.

Look into other lifestyle factors

Once you have taken the time and dedication to get yourself following the rules of the Paleo diet, make sure you are also incorporating other healthy habits that will ensure that you feel your absolute best, such as plenty of exercises, sleep, stress management, and time out in the sun soaking up Vitamin D.

Chapter 3: The Top 5 Paleo Mistakes

Making the decision to switch to the way our ancestors ate is one of the best things you can do for your health and well-being. Many folks spend years of time trying out new "fad" diets, only to be left disappointed after valuable time was wasted counting calories and eating minimal, not so yummy meals. In fact, many people feel sicker and even older when attempting the new trends. If you are tired of chasing trends and really want to make a difference in your personal life, then you will find that choosing to go on the Paleo diet is one of the best choices you will make!

The Paleo diet does go against much of the common nutritional advice we all receive as we grow up. The first thing one must remember when trying out any diet, let alone the Paleo, is to have an open mind, for this is the first real stride that is taken in order to feel better.

This chapter is here to inform newbies that are thinking or just started the process of incorporating the Paleo diet into their lives about the most common mistakes that almost everyone makes while on it. I deem this chapter highly crucial to your success on this diet. Once people become knowledgeable of these mistakes, it is easier to avoid them.

Quitting Too Soon

When people conduct themselves on the Paleo diet properly, it can provide those great benefits for years to come. But like changing anything in life, the first few weeks are going to be tough. You will crash, and you will end up feeling more tired than before since your body is getting used to the new form of fuel you are providing it. Creating and sticking to new habits can be challenging physically, so be prepared to not feel your absolute best for a few weeks. Just like drug and alcohol addicts must rid their bodies of the toxins these substances have in them, you are ridding yourself of all the bad things that grains and sugars have in them, for they are just as addictive.

And don't fool yourself, one of the biggest obstacles on any diet is the challenges that come with a social life. You will get a weird look from friends, family, and coworkers. They will more than likely push you back to eating the same old stuff you did before.

It is natural to not be able to figure out everything in the first few weeks, so don't put yourself down. Just take action and ensure that you are making small changes along the journey to a better you! Sticking to it, no matter how hard it gets, will help you to reap major benefits later on. Whatever you do, do not just give up after a mere few weeks.

Failure to Plan

Changing the entire perspective of your everyday diet is an investment to your life, both mentally and physically. You will get more out of life, but in order to achieve this, you must be willing to put in the hard work to get there first. Like you have read, the first few weeks are inevitably going to be challenging. You must push away and avoid foods you are not allowed to eat. You may even be making meals for yourself for the first time in a while or ever.

I am sure you have questions, such as how you will eat dinner if you have to stay at work late, or what happens when you become hungry as you are out and about running errands. These certainly are good questions to consider. This is why is it vital to come up with a plan that will help you to successfully stick to the Paleo diet. With a plan comes the peace of mind that it will be a bit easier to actually succeed on this new diet plan. Yes, you will have to tweak things as you go along, but it is definitely worth it in the long run.

Thinking of the Paleo as a "Detox Diet"

The list of foods that you must avoid while on the Paleo diet can seem rather daunting, especially to beginners. Many newbies hone in on what not to eat and rid themselves of rather than what they should be consuming. They get in the mindset that this diet is more of a detox rather than an entirely new and healthier lifestyle.

If you only worry yourself over the foods you must cut out of your everyday diet, you are paving the way for disaster to strike. You will end up not consuming enough calories since you are not actually considering the additional fats and proteins you need to be eating. This means you end up tired and hungry, which fuels your irritation. If you want to really change your lifestyle in regards to your diet, this is no place to be. So remember, the Paleo diet is not a detox, but it is all about making the right food decisions. Don't view it as just trying to constantly avoid food.

Constantly Aiming for Perfection

Many folks who start their journey on the Paleo diet get it stuck in their mind that this diet is an "all or nothing" sort of deal.

They then tend to beat themselves up when they shove a few French fries in their face. Or once they succumb to one or two cravings of sugars and carbs, they tell themselves that this diet is just not for them.

It is important to get in the mindset that any type of progress is the goal you should strive for, not absolute perfection. Every single good decision you make is a step in the right direction. Eating well for the majority of the day and then having some ice cream at the end is much better than eating badly all day and then having ice cream. "Perfectly Paleo" should be seen as an ideal, not as a requirement. Make the best choices you can at the time with what you have. But do not beat yourself up if you get off track a few times. Just hold your head high and pick up where you left off, and continue to trudge forward. This is a good thing to remember, for it is the only way to prosperous long-term success.

Being Scared of Carbs

Carbohydrates are seen as evil things by many people, especially the individuals who try out every single new diet fad but find no success. Low-carb diets are great ways to lose weight and become healthier, but many people take the low-carb mindset too far. People tend to hone in on the fact that they should "avoid" carbs altogether, even ones that come from fruits and veggies.

All this manages to do is leave you feeling hunger pangs all the time if you are not replacing those carbs with lots of healthy fats and proteins. This is even more challenging for those that like to work out a lot or work strenuous jobs. It is much easier to go Paleo if they added healthy carbs to make up the highly physical demands their body requires them to perform.

The amount of carbs each person needs varies. If you are on the Paleo diet and constantly feel hungry, tired, or just not like yourself, try incorporating some healthy carbs into the mix. This could be just the fix you need in order to feel great while on the Paleo diet.

(Enjoying this book so far? I'd love to see your opinion on Amazon. Scan QR code below to leave a review)

Chapter 4: Paleo Diet Plan for Successful Weight Loss

The basis of the Paleo diet is taking a hard look at the hunter and gather tendencies that our ancestors had to have to thrive and survive. Our ancestors did not have access to grocery stores that were packed with consumables that could be popped in the microwave. Our genetics are the same as our cavemen counterparts, but they were free from diseases like heart disease, diabetes, and obesity. Why? Because their diets were made up of all-natural eats, rather than highly-processed foods full of carbs and excess sugars.

The Paleo diet has been proven to lead to significant weight loss without the hassle of counting calories and packing foods into portion control containers. It has also been shown to lead to major improvements in health.

One of the coolest things about the Paleo diet is that there is not necessarily one way to eat. Our Paleolithic ancestors ate a variety of things, all dependent on what resources they had available at the time. There were times that they ate low-carb diets that were high in animal fats and proteins, while other times they ate diets high in carbs that consisted of plants.

Planning on the Paleo can be rather challenging, so here are a few tips to remember:

- Pile half your plate with vegetables.
- Have 1-2 palm-sized servings of animal proteins.

- Incorporate some sort of healthy fat, like coconut or olive oil.
- Optional: include some nuts, fruits, and starchy vegetables.

For all the eager beginners that wish to start the Paleo diet, the remainder of this chapter outlines a simple and basic 1-week diet plan that aims to aid in weight loss.

One Week Paleo Diet Plan

Monday

- **Breakfast** – Veggies and eggs, fried up in coconut oil. 1 piece of fruit
- **Lunch** – Chicken salad with olive oil. 1 handful nuts.
- **Dinner** – Burger with no bun, fried in butter with veggies and salsa

Tuesday

- **Breakfast** – Eggs and bacon. 1 piece of fruit.
- **Lunch** – Leftover burgers from the evening before.
- **Dinner** – Salmon fried in butter. Veggies.

Wednesday

- **Breakfast** – Leftover meat and veggies from the evening before.
- **Lunch** – Sandwich with lettuce serving as bread. Serve with meat and veggies.
- **Dinner** – Ground beef stir-fry with veggies. 1 handful berries.

Thursday

- **Breakfast** – Eggs and 1 piece of fruit.
- **Lunch** – Leftover stir-fry from the evening before. 1 handful nuts.
- **Dinner** Fried pork with veggies

Friday

- **Breakfast** – Eggs and veggies, fried in coconut oil.
- **Lunch** – Chicken salad with olive oil. 1 handful of nuts.
- **Dinner** – Steak with veggies and sweet potatoes

Saturday

- **Breakfast** – Bacon and eggs. 1 piece of fruit
- **Lunch** – Leftover steak and veggies from the evening before.
- **Dinner** – Baked salmon with veggies and avocado.

Sunday

- **Breakfast** – Leftover meat and veggies from evening before.
- **Lunch** – Sandwich with lettuce leaves serving as bread. Served with fresh veggies.
- **Dinner** – Grilled chicken wings with veggies and salsa.

Making Restaurant Meals More Paleo

There are going to be times that come up that you have to eat out at restaurants. Here are a few pointers into helping make restaurant meals more Paleo based:

- Ask to have your food cooked in coconut or olive oil.
- Get extra veggies instead of rice or bread as sides.
- Order fish-based or a meat-based dish.

Simple Paleo Snacks

There is no reason to eat more than three meals per day, but sometimes you will get hungry in-between meals. So here is a list of simple snacks to curb those bad cravings you may get:

- Homemade beef jerky
- Bowl of berries with coconut cream
- Apple slices with almond butter
- Leftover from evening before
- Handful of nuts
- Piece of fruit
- Hard-boiled eggs
- Baby carrots

Chapter 5: Paleo Diet Tips and Tricks

The Paleo diet can inevitably present beginners with struggles and obstacles to overcome. In order to have the best chance possible to really be successful, this chapter was written with a variety of tips and tricks that will help to move the scales to your favor. All of these pointers are made to make transitioning into the Paleo diet as painless as it possibly can be!

- Eat the entire egg – Put a conclusion to the egg white versus egg yolk wrangle about and simply eat the darn things. Imagining Paleo man isolating their eggs is practically entertaining. A large portion of the supplements originate from the yolk, and you'll be bending over the measure of protein by going entirety.

- Cave dwellers moved, you ought to as well – Our present-day way of life bears us the solace of sitting in one place throughout the day, regardless of whether that is an office seat, auto seat, or couch. How about we wind the clock back a couple of dozen centuries and do what we did while being relaxed wasn't a choice. The more you move the better you'll feel and the positive cycle will proceed.

- Plan ahead – Don't give an attack of craving sneak a chance up on you and make you get wrecked from your Paleo way. Suspect getting ravenous, and look forward to your day to check whether there are any circumstances or occasions where you'll wind up in a position to swindle. Get ready dinners and snacks that will hold you over until the point that your next feast time.

- Purchase more vegetables – Every time you go to the store make it a propensity to stack up on vegetables. Veggies are the way to influencing Paleo to work, and not eating enough of them is the primary reason individuals don't get comes about. There's a decent amount of meat eaten on Paleo, yet the enchantment is in getting enough vegetables.

- Don't go it alone– Cavemen lived in tight weave groups, chasing and assembling in gatherings and moving together to discover better assets. It's best to do Paleo with someone else, and in any event, you'll need to get the help of your family and companions.

- Organic products are not the adversary – While the natural product is not a point of convergence of the Paleo abstain from food, it's additionally not your foe, so don't treat it like it will send you off track. Having a serving of natural product every day will give you cancer prevention agents, additional fiber, and an essence of something sweet.

- It's OK to be ravenous in some cases – It's flawlessly normal to get eager, be satisfied for a little while, and after that get ravenous once more. Try not to fear being ravenous, it's great to have a solid hunger before your dinners. Your yearning level dependably reveals to you something about what's new with your body, so hear it out.

- Nothing beats effortlessness – Keeping things straightforward on the Paleo count calories is basic on the off chance that you need to succeed. Early man was compelled to keep it basic, yet present-day man needs to intentionally take things back to a more straightforward time. The more you entangle a feast the less Paleo it is.

- Investigate your numerous alternatives – If you ever wind up believing that the Paleo eat less is prohibitive, take a look at yourself and recollect that there are a lot of various alternatives accessible to you. Because you won't be eating the things you used to, similar to dairy, grains, and sugar, you can at present have an adjusted and changed eating regimen that fulfills.

- Go outside – There's no denying that Paleolithic man spends an incredible lion's share of his chance outside. That is a conspicuous difference to the way we spend our days now, so take each risk you get the opportunity to go outside and get collective with nature.

- Supplant, don't control – Diets that deny you to have a specific kind of nourishment, similar to sweets or chocolate, are limited. You'll need to start supplanting unapproved nourishments with appropriate substitutes. To influence this truly simple we to have 27 Paleo Substitutions so you can see a fast "utilize this, not" Paleo control.

- Nobody needs to concur with you – It won't be well before somebody tags along and lets you know the Paleo abstain from food is senseless. That is OK on the grounds that there's just a single individual that needs necessities to get ready regarding the theory: You.

- Purchase natural – Whenever conceivable, settle on natural create. This basically takes nourishment back to a period when pesticides and herbicides weren't utilized to develop sustenance, and recoveries your body from these lethal chemicals.

- Rest more – Sleep is so imperative to your general prosperity that you'll need to ensure you're getting enough of it at the correct time. Go into the circadian beat of life and calendar your wake up and rest times as indicated by the regular rhythms your body experiences.

- Unplug – It's so natural to spend a large portion of the day on a cell phone or PC, yet it's not what we were intended to do. Split far from LCD screens for no less than an hour a day to give your eyes a rest and live more normally.

- Lift weights – keeping in mind the end goal to get a mountain man's body you will need to lift like one. Lift overwhelming weights with low reps to construct the kind of physical make-up that could cut down a mastodon. For a stone age woman's body concentrate on bodyweight practices that include the entire body immediately.

- Get daylight – If you're getting outside more this conceivable won't be an issue. Simply ensure that you are getting some sun presentation on exposed skin without consuming yourself. The expansion in Vitamin D will help your body gigantically.

- Search for advance in all parts of your life – If you're doing Paleo to shed pounds, remember to watch your life in general and see that it's affecting all that you do. You may see a change by the way you feel, you'll stretch less, connections will enhance, and work execution will increment.

- Get acquainted with ghee – This is one wellspring of fat that you can use on Paleo. It's produced using spread yet has been "illuminated" by having the greater part of the debasements expelled from it. Its rich flavor improves pretty much anything taste.

- Get out your crock pot – Time to begin a relationship with your Crock Pot. It's a dependable approach to make Paleo suppers without spending a cluster of time keeping an eye on nourishment at the stove. It's so natural to put a supper on in the morning and make them sit tight for you when you return home for supper.

- Be willing to learn – There's constantly more to find with Paleo, and a few masters give the logical premise to why it works. Regardless of how far down the rabbit opening you need to go, there will dependably be new formulas, tips, and data accessible to take in and apply to your life.

- Be tolerant with yourself – Following the Paleo count calories is a procedure, so don't be too hard on yourself on the off chance that you experience difficulty adhering to it at the very begin. It can be difficult to surrender the things that you've developed so used to eating, and embrace another, outside method for eating.

- Try fasting – Our Paleo predecessors wouldn't have had 3 square dinners a day following a seeker gatherer way of life. Discontinuous fasting has been appeared to help with fat misfortune and copies the devour and starvation lifestyle that was the standard.

- Stock up on Paleo sustenance – A cooler brimming with Paleo sustenance is an incredible sight, and it is a vital approach to give your mind the flag that you aren't starving, and that there's bounty to eat. It likewise improves you prepared to pursue Paleo formulas on the web and have the capacity to take after along.

- Perceive how you like organ meats – They may not sound excessively engaging at to start with, but rather they don't taste vastly different than the meats you're accustomed to eating, it's all the more a mental thing knowing you're eating organ meats. These are stacked with vitamins and minerals and are extremely in accordance with hereditary eating.

- Search for things to get simpler as you come – Beginning is the hardest part. In the event that you can endure the main month of Paleo, you'll get to the guaranteed arrive. That is the reason you'll see 3-week and 30-day Paleo challenges since it truly will be a test to stick to it impeccably for a month.

- Figure out how to like scraps – Leftovers are a method for keeping things basic, and of living all the more proficiently on the grounds that you're getting two suppers out of the time it takes to set one up.

- Keep in mind play time – It's anything but difficult to get excessively genuine about it all and neglect to invest significant time to play. Have a ton of fun every day, play a game, play a prepackaged game, get included with others and lose yourself at the time.

- Devour solid fat each day – The Standard American Diet incorporates barely any solid fat. Rectify this unevenness by ensuring you eat avocados, nuts, seeds, and solid oils to get the monounsaturated and polyunsaturated fat into your life.

- Enhance your cooking – You'll likely be doing significantly more cooking on Paleo than you ever have before on the grounds that it's the main way you can have finish quality control of your suppers. Show signs of improvement at cooking and you'll have a superior and more charming time on Paleo.

- Drink a lot of water – Don't neglect to drink your water while on Paleo. Ensure it's very much purged and oppose the compulsion to include fluid sweeteners that have turned out to be prevalent lately.

- Disregard what you think about "eating methodologies" – Paleo doesn't subscribe to the greater part of the principles and controls that huge numbers of the most renowned eating regimen designs do. No compelling reason to tally carbs, calories, focuses, or to measure yourself. Eat genuine sustenance and utilize the mirror and how you feel to gaze at your progress.

- Line yourself up – Make beyond any doubt that your body is in line with the goal that it's legitimately working. This may involve doing day by day activities or seeing a chiropractor in case you're crooked, however, it will have an immense effect in case you're right now broken in your developments.

- Prepare with interims – Interval preparing is a more viable approach to do cardio, and it takes advantage of our inborn need to feel a burst of adrenaline as we keep running as quickly as possible. Attempt interims where you dash for 30 seconds and run softly for 30 seconds to a moment.

- Hold some present-day enhancements – There's no compelling reason to live precisely like a Stone Age man with a specific end goal to receive the rewards. Utilize a blender to mix up smoothies, utilize your auto to get you around, and utilize your telephone and PC to stay in contact with friends and family. Be that as it may, don't give it a chance to make you languid.

- Try things out first – With such a large number of various vegetables accessible, numerous that you might not have attempted some time recently, you might be enticed to turn your nose up at some of them. In any case, make certain to attempt them first before deciding. You may find another sustenance that you cherish and never knew it existed.

- Alter your eatery orders – Many of the eatery things you'll discover are practically Paleo yet not exactly. Make certain to give clear directions to the server with the goal that your feast does exclude any grains or dairy. Swap in an additional side of veggies for the dull sides served at generally eateries.

- Have your fair treats – You don't have to pass on dessert insofar as you've made yourself a Paleo dessert. This program is not a trial of self-discipline or a method for influencing you to ache for every one of the things you used to have, it's tied in with taking in another method for eating.

- Build up your 7 go-to suppers – Try the same number of Paleo supper formulas as it takes to gather 7 distinct meals that you an) affection b) are anything but difficult to make c) you wouldn't see any problems with having on a week after week premise. You would then be able to pivot them out and have something else each night of the week. The same should be possible for breakfast and lunch and you'll have a wide range of everyday blends to work with.

- Parity your suppers – Many outcasts trust Paleo is about everything you-can-eat bacon or porterhouse steaks at each dinner. While protein servings are a factor in Paleo, you need to eat adjusted dinners that have similarly the same number of vegetables as meat on the plate. On the off chance that you skew, skew towards the side of more veggies.

- Get insightful about nourishment marks – Learn how to peruse sustenance names and get acquainted with the distinctive names for things like MSG and the diverse fake sweeteners. Or, on the other hand, make it super basic and eat sustenance that doesn't accompany "Nourishment" names.

- Utilize coconut oil for cooking and preparing – Turn a hard of hearing ear to the verbal confrontation on coconut oil and begin utilizing it to cook with. It likewise makes an awesome showing with regards to in heated products, and they'll turn out tasting superior to anything the locally acquired stuff with no flour or sugar utilized.

- Consider purging before going Paleo – A detoxing purify is a smart thought in case you will begin Paleo in light of the fact that it will make a wedge between how you used to eat and how you'll eat starting now and into the foreseeable future. It cleanses the body of some developed poisons and makes the Paleo method for eating more successful.

- At the point when the climate grants, start up the flame broil – Next, to a Crock-Pot, your grill flame broil is the following nearest cooking device to impersonate the Stone Age man method for cooking. Attempt a flame-broiled chicken bosom or salmon loaded with barbecued asparagus lances and Portobello mushroom tops.

- Take a world visit in your kitchen – You can test the distinctive foods of the world while never leaving your home. Paleo welcomes you to utilize seasonings and flavors outside of your usual range of familiarity. Your taste buds will bless your heart.

- In case you will cheat, cheat right – If you feel a cheat supper developing, make it a decent one that tends to your most requesting yearnings. At that point get appropriate back on track and don't pummel yourself about it. Invest considerably more energy to make adjusted suppers and utilize substitutions so you don't motivate longings, to begin with.

- Get a predator's mindset – Reclaiming the attitude of a predator is one approach to get into the Paleo outlook. People didn't generally have simple access to nourishment, we needed to get off our bottoms and go pursue it down. You don't have to chase your nourishment, simply have that same zeal with regards to setting up your sustenance as opposed to influencing it to feel like a drag.

- Try not to disparage the energy of smoothies – You can participate on the smoothie furor clearing the country. Simply make sure to utilize qualified Paleo smoothie formulas so you keep it dairy-free and sound. Cancer prevention agents ahoy!

- If all else fails, have salmon – Stuck for a supper thought? Salmon is a flavorful fish that gets suggested by well-being advocates no matter how you look at it. The omega-3s it contains are a critical piece of Paleo well-being and prosperity.

- Flour can be your companion – If it arrives in a crate and has flour in the fixings show, it's not your companion. On the off chance that you utilize almond flour or coconut flour you'll be getting included fiber and a comparable taste and surface. Banishing universally handy flour from your eating routine is sufficient to get results and one a player in the greater Paleo picture.

- Be the weirdo in social circumstances – It's superbly adequate to be the one that isn't drinking at a bar, or the one that conveys their lunch to work, or the one that gives additional requests to the server at an eatery. You are accomplishing something other than what's expected, and you'll get diverse outcomes as a result of it.

- Take control of caffeine – Assess whether caffeine is having its way with you, or you're having your way with it. In the event that you just can't live without it, you might need to consider surrendering it for a little while and afterward coming back to it just now and again.

- Take up a game – Going on Paleo is the ideal time to take up a game. Paleo is a standout amongst other eating regimens to take after for competitors, and regardless of what you start up, you'll profit by the protein and supplements Paleo gives.

- Never be without recipes – Surround yourself with a lot of assets for Paleo formulas. You'll need them all readily available so you're not wasting your time when it comes time to choose what to eat. Nowadays you're in luckiness, on the grounds that there are a lot of Paleo formula online journals and books to browse with heaps of flavorful formulas.

Chapter 6: Body Healing on the Paleo Diet

As you have read so far, the Paleolithic diet has many great benefits, but to some, that may not be enough to make the switch. Did you know that a diet engulfed in grains, carbohydrates, sugars, and unhealthy oils can actually lead to a substantial amount of health issues down the line? Diets rich in these not so great eats can lead to a leaky gut, autoimmune disorders, chronic fatigue, inflammatory bowel disease, rashes, diabetes, mental disorders, and a wide array of other issues as well. Now that just doesn't sound great at all, does it? This doesn't even take into account all of the prescription and antibiotic drugs that we utilize on an almost daily basis. All of these things can really throw your body's natural rhythms out of whack.

If you have yet to adopt the Paleo diet, there is a very good chance that your insides are allowing toxins right into the bloodstream, which prevents nutrients from getting to where they need to go, even if you are one that eats relatively healthy.

That is one of the most beneficial aspects of the Paleo diet, the fact that is aids in the health of many areas of the insides of our bodies. The Paleo diet is a major step in restoring the equilibrium of our inner selves, which leads us to feeling a heck of a lot better than we may already feel!

Healing the Gut

Each and everything that we devour is sent to your stomach and gut, and all things have a somewhat different reaction. There are certain edibles that will increase the permeability of our gut, which if done long-term, can allow digest food particles into the bloodstream, which results in an immune response. This is how autoimmune disorders can develop. On the Paleo diet, you are already avoiding the list of foods below, which is one of the reasons it is so darn beneficial in creating a better balance of health. Here are the foods responsible for a lack of healing in your gut:

- Grains
- Excess of carbs
- Alcohol
- Caffeine
- Unhealthy oils
- Sugars
- Dairy
- Legumes

By taking these foods out of your diet, you have a better chance to reduce the inflammation that can occur in the stomach and gut, which helps to restore its overall health.

Foods that are enriched with probiotics are essential for gut health. Our gut is a home for over 100 trillion organisms, which is why certain foods really disrupt its natural flow. The following foods are rich in these important probiotics and should be consumed on a regular basis:

- Dairy-free supplements
- Kombucha
- Fermented veggies, like kimchi and sauerkraut

Celebrities that Utilize the Paleo Diet

Celebrities, as we all know, are best known for being physically fit. This is because they easily have access to nutritionists and personal trainers, who encourage them to eat a more Paleolithic-based diet. Below is a list of renowned individuals that swear by the Paleo diet in order to keep their health in check:

- Miley Cyrus
- Megan Fox
- Eva LaRue
- Jimmy Fallon
- Commando Steve
- Gwyneth Paltrow
- Tom Jones
- Jessica Biel
- Jack Osbourne

Athletes on the Paleo

Athletes need to look and feel their best in order to be in the physical condition that is required of them to be successful. This is why a large majority of the most famous athletes incorporate Paleolithic methods into their everyday diets. Here are a few:

- Dwight Howard
- Novak Djokovic
- Abe Wagner
- Iris Lazz
- Kelly Slater
- Amanda Beard
- Josh Welburn
- Greg Parnham
- The entire Lakers Basketball Team
- Kobe Bryant
- LeBron James
- Carol Nichols

Chapter 7: Paleo Breakfast Recipes

Apple Muffins

What's in it:

- 1 ¼ C. granny smith apple chunks
- ½ C. grated granny smith apples
- 2 tsp. vanilla extract
- 1/3 C. maple syrup
- 5 tbsp. melted coconut oil
- 2 eggs
- ¼ tsp. ground nutmeg
- 1 tbsp. ground cinnamon
- ¼ tsp. salt
- ½ tsp. baking soda
- 2 ½ tbsp. coconut flour
- 1 ¼ C. blanched almond flour

How it's made:

- Ensure the oven is preheated to 350 degrees. Use the muffin liners to line a muffin tin.
- Mix all the dry components together then set aside.
- Mix the syrup, vanilla, oil, and eggs together. Then mix the dry mixture till combined.
- Fold in the grated apples then mix the chopped apples.
- Pour batter into liners, fill them ¾+ of the way full.
- Bake for 23-35 minutes.
- Allow to cool for 5 minutes and remove from the muffin tin. Let the muffins cool completely.

Turkey and Egg Breakfast Casserole

What's in it:

- Pepper and salt
- 1 C. baby spinach
- 1 sweet potato (peeled/thinly sliced)
- 12 eggs
- ½ tsp. chili powder
- 1 pound ground turkey
- 1 tbsp. coconut oil + more for coating pan

Other Toppings:

- Tomatoes
- Diced onions
- Asparagus

How it's made:

- Ensure the oven is preheated to 375 degrees. With the coconut oil, grease a 9x9 pan.
- Warm up 1 tbsp coconut oil in a pan. Once melted, add the turkey. Season with pepper, salt, and chili powder then cook till browned.
- Peel the sweet potato as turkey cooks and slice thinly.
- Line the bottom of the dish with the potatoes.
- Beat the eggs and season with pepper and salt.
- Pour the turkey and eggs over top of the potatoes. Layer the spinach over top, as well as any other toppings you wish to incorporate.
- Cook for 35-40 minutes till the edges start to brown and the casserole is firm.

Paleo Pancakes

What's in it:

- 1 tsp. vanilla extract
- 1 tsp. cinnamon
- 1 tbsp. coconut flour
- 2 eggs
- 1 banana

Toppings:

- Maple syrup
- Fruit of choice
- Dark chocolate chips

How it's made:

- Mash up the banana, and then mix the vanilla, cinnamon, coconut flour, and eggs. Combine well.
- Warm up a pan.
- Pour the batter into even sized pancakes. Sprinkle with toppings of choice into cakes.
- Cook for 2-4 minutes. Flip and cook the other side for 2 minutes.
- Drizzle with syrup and enjoy!

Bacon Pancakes

What's in it:

- Dash of sea salt
- ¼ tsp. baking soda
- 2/3 C. unsweetened coconut milk
- 2 tbsp. melted coconut oil
- 2 eggs
- ¼ C. coconut flour
- 4 strips no-sugar-added/uncured bacon
- Ghee (to cook with)

How it's made:

- Warm up a griddle then cook the bacon till crisp. Set to the side.
- Whisk the eggs, coconut oil, and coconut milk together. Then mix the baking soda, sea salt, and coconut flour till smooth.
- Melt a tbsp of ghee in griddle. Pour batter onto griddle in strip form. Put a piece of bacon in each strip and drizzle more batter on top.
- Cook for 4-5 minutes till golden.
- Flip and then cook another 4-5 minutes.
- Serve with pure maple syrup.

Turkey Apple Breakfast Hash

What's in it:

Meat:

- Sea salt
- ½ tsp. cinnamon
- ½ tsp. dried thyme
- 1 tbsp. coconut oil
- 1 pound ground turkey

Hash:

- ½ tsp. dried thyme
- ½ tsp. turmeric
- ½ tsp. garlic powder
- ¾ tsp. powdered ginger
- 2 C. spinach
- 1 peeled/cored/chopped apple
- 2 C. frozen butternut squash
- ½ C. shredded carrots
- 1 large zucchini
- 1 onion
- 1 tbsp. coconut oil
- Sea salt

How it's made:

- Warm up a tbsp coconut oil, and then add the turkey. Cook till browned. Season with sea salt, thyme, and cinnamon. Transfer to the plate.

- Pour remaining coconut oil into the skillet and sauté onion 2-3 minutes till soft.
- Pour the squash, apple, carrots, and zucchini into the onion, cook 4-5 minutes till soft.
- Stir in the spinach till wilted.
- Add the turkey, seasonings, and salt then turn the heat off.
- Eat right out of the skillet or allow to cool and chill, eat throughout the week.

Sweet Potato Waffle Breakfast Sandwich

What's in it:

- ½ sliced avocado
- 1 C. chopped kale
- 1 tsp. oil + more for waffle iron/frying pan
- 1/8 tsp. garlic salt
- 1/8 tsp. paprika
- ¼ tsp. cumin
- 1 uncooked skinned/grated sweet potato
- 2 eggs
- Pepper and salt

What's in it:

- Warm up the waffle iron then grease liberally.
- Whisk the eggs then add the grated sweet potato along with seasonings and 1 tsp of oil. Mix thoroughly.
- Pack a sweet potato mixture into the iron. Press the iron gently and cook for 4-5 minutes till lightly golden.

- Warm up oil in a pan and then sauté kale for 3-4 minutes till crisp.
  Fry the egg in the same pan.
- When the sweet potato waffle is ready, remove with a butter knife and put on a plate. Place the avocado slices, fried egg, and kale on top. Season with pepper and salt. Enjoy!

<u>Cinnamon Sugar Pumpkin Donut Holes</u>

What's in it:

Donut Holes:

- 2 tsp. vanilla extract
- ½ C. canned pumpkin puree
- 2 tbsp. coconut sugar
- ½ C. maple syrup
- 7 tbsp. unsalted butter
- 4 eggs
- ¼ tsp. salt
- 3 ½ tsp. pumpkin pie spice
- 1 ¼ tsp. baking soda
- ¾ C. almond flour
- ½ C. coconut flour

Cinnamon Sugar:

- 1 ½ tsp. ground cinnamon
- 1/3 C. coconut sugar

How it's made:

- Ensure the oven is preheated to 350 degrees. With the muffin liners, line a muffin pan.
- Mix all the dry components of donut holes together.
- Mix together all the wet components of donut holes.
- Incorporate the wet and dry mixtures together, combining well.
- Pour the batter into the muffin tin, filling till almost full.
- Bake for 11-13 minutes.
- Mix the cinnamon and sugar together in a small bowl. When ready to serve, roll donut holes in cinnamon sugar.

Chapter 8: Paleo Lunch Recipes

Bacon Scallion Chicken Salad

What's in it:

- Pepper and salt
- ½ tsp. garlic powder
- ½ C. Paleo-friendly mayo
- 2 scallions
- ½ C. green onions
- 8 slices nitrate-free bacon
- 1 pound boneless skinless chicken breasts

How it's made:

- Chop the bacon into pieces then brown till crisp.
- Drain the bacon on paper towels and save the bacon fat that remains in the pan.
- Pound the chicken till its ½ inch thick then cut in half.
- Sprinkle the chicken with garlic, pepper, and salt and place in the pan with the bacon fat. Cook for 2-3 minutes till insides are no longer pink.
- Place the cooked chicken in a bowl and chill till cooled.
- Chop the chicken into pieces and toss with mayo, scallions, and bacon.
- Season with pepper and salt to reach the desired taste.

Chicken and Zucchini Poppers

What's in it:

- ½ tsp. pepper
- 1 tsp. salt
- 1 clove of garlic
- 3-4 tbsp. minced cilantro
- 2-3 sliced green onions
- 2 C. grated zucchini
- 1 pound ground chicken breast
- Olive oil or ghee

How it's made:

- Toss together the pepper, salt, garlic, cilantro, green onion, zucchini, and chicken together.
- Warm up the oil. Create balls out of the chicken mixture and place in a pan then cook for 8-10 minutes. Flip and cook another for 4-5 minutes till golden brown.
- Serve with guacamole, your favorite dip, or salsa. Enjoy!

Buffalo Chicken Celery Sticks

What's in it:

- 6 celery stalks (cut in half to make 12)
- 3 tbsp. buffalo wing sauce
- ¼ tsp. pepper and salt
- ½ tsp. garlic powder
- ¼ C. mayo
- 2 C. shredded chicken
- Chopped chives, garnish

How it's made:

- Combine the buffalo wing sauce, salt, pepper, garlic powder, mayo, and chicken together.
- Fill each piece of celery with the chicken mixture. Sprinkle with chopped chives.

BBQ Chicken and Roasted Sweet Potato Bowls

What's in it:

- Salt
- ½ C. BBQ sauce
- 1 pound boneless skinless chicken breasts
- 1 head broccoli
- ½ tsp. chipotle powder
- ½ tsp. garlic powder
- ½ tsp. salt
- 2 tbsp. olive oil
- 1 yellow onion
- 2 sweet potatoes

How it's made:

- Ensure the oven is preheated to 400 degrees.
- Peel and chop the potatoes into ½" chunks. Chop the onion into pieces.
- On a lined baking sheet, pour the sweet potatoes and onions on. Toss with a tbsp of olive oil, ¼ tsp salt, garlic powder, and chipotle powder. Toss well and bake for 20 minutes.
- Push the potatoes to one side of the pan then add broccoli and toss with olive oil and remaining salt. Add the chicken breasts, and brush with a ¼ cup of the BBQ

sauce. Bake for another 15-20 minutes till the chicken is completely cooked.
- Take off the pan and shred the chicken. Toss with the remaining BBQ sauce.
- Add to the bowls with roasted veggies.

Strawberry Mango Salad with Chicken

What's in it:

Strawberry Poppy Seed Dressing:

- ½ C. strawberries
- ¼ C. honey
- 1/3 C. champagne vinegar
- ½ C. olive oil
- 1 tbsp. poppy seeds
- ¼ tsp. salt

Mango Salad:

- 1 C. roasted/sliced almonds
- 1 chopped avocado
- 1 C. chopped strawberries
- 1 chopped mango
- 2 8-ounce chopped/cooked chicken breasts
- 8 C. baby greens

How it's made:

- To make the dressing, mix together all the dressing components in a blender till smooth.
- To make the salad, combine all the salad components together. Then toss with dressing. Serve right away.

Plantain Carnitas Nachos

What's in it:

- Juice of ½ lime
- 1 tsp. sea salt
- 2 tbsp. coconut oil
- 3 tbsp. cilantro
- ¼ C. red onion
- 2 servings avocado lime sauce
- 2 servings pork carnitas
- 2 green sliced plantains

How it's made:

- Warm up a coconut oil in a pan.
- When melted, add the plantain slices.
- Cook till soft and lightly browned.
- Take off heat, and mash them with the bottom of a glass to flatten them.
- Put flattened plantains back in the oil then cook till crisp.
- Layer plantains with lime sauce, cilantro, red onion, and carnitas.
- Top with more lime if you want to.

Crunchy Crusted Coconut Chicken

What's in it:

- Pepper and salt
- 1 C. shredded coconut
- 2 eggs
- 2 chicken breasts

How it's made:

- Cut the chicken up into strips, then beat them till they are an even thickness.
- Then whisk then eggs.
- Put the shredded coconut in a separate bowl from eggs.
- Drop the chicken into the eggs then into the coconut.
- Repeat till all the chicken is coated.
- Warm up the oil in a pan, then add the coated chicken.
- Cook for 3-5 minutes on each side till golden brown.

Chapter 9: Paleo Dinner Recipes

Tomato Basil Turkey Meatloaf

What's in it:

- 1 tsp. salt
- 1 tsp. garlic powder
- 1 egg
- 3 tbsp. chopped basil
- 2 tbsp. tomato paste
- ¼ C. almond flour
- 1 pound ground turkey

Topping:

- Pinch of salt
- 1 tbsp. chopped basil
- 1 tbsp. apple cider vinegar
- ¼ C. chopped tomatoes

How it's made:

- Ensure the oven is preheated to 400 degrees.
- Mix all of the meatloaf components together till well combined.
  Ball up the mixture and form into a loaf shape on a lined baking sheet.
- Mix all of the topping components together and then spoon over top of the meatloaf.
- Bake for 30 minutes.

Cilantro Lime Chicken with Avocado Salsa

What's in it:

Chicken:

- ¼ tsp. salt
- ½ tsp. ground cumin
- ¼ C. cilantro
- 2 tbsp. olive oil
- ¼ C. lime juice
- 1 ½ pounds boneless chicken breast

Avocado Salsa:

- Salt
- 1 minced clove garlic
- ½ tsp. red pepper flakes
- ½ tsp. red wine vinegar
- 3 tbsp. lime juice
- ½ C. diced cilantro
- 4 diced avocados

How it's made:

- Whisk the salt, cumin, cilantro, olive oil, and lime juice together.
- Put the chicken into a Ziploc bag and pour the marinade. Allow to mix for 15 minutes.
- Heat up the grill. Put the chicken on the grill then cook each side for 4-6 minutes. Allow to sit.
- To make the salsa, mix all the salsa components together, and toss gently to incorporate.
- Top the chicken with salsa and serve!

Italian Style Spaghetti Squash Bake

What's in it:

Spaghetti Squash:

- ½ tsp. pepper and salt
- 2 tsp. extra-virgin olive oil
- 1 spaghetti squash

Other components:

- ½ tsp. pepper and salt
- 1 tbsp. garlic powder
- ½ tsp. red pepper flakes
- 1 ½ tbsp. Italian seasoning
- 1 egg
- 1 C. tomato sauce
- 1 pound boneless chicken breasts
- 3 handfuls spinach
- 1 crushed clove garlic
- 1 tsp. extra-virgin olive oil

How it's made:

- Ensure the oven is preheated to 375 degrees.
- Cut the squash in half and then scoop out seeds. Sprinkle with pepper, salt, and olive oil.
- With a parchment paper, line a baking sheet.
- Place squash face down on the sheet and add ¼ cup of water. Bake for 30 minutes till squash is fork-tender. Allow to cool.

- When cooled, scrape squash using a fork then place in a bowl.
- Warm up the oil and sauté the garlic. Add the spinach, sautéing till wilted.
- Add the cheese, egg, tomato sauce, shredded chicken, garlic, and spinach mixture with the shredded squash. Combine well.
- Pour into a baking dish and sprinkle with parmesan and red pepper flakes.
- Bake for 10 minutes then broil 3-5 minutes till cheese is bubbly and browned.

Asparagus Sweet Potato Chicken Skillet

What's in it:

- ½ tsp. crushed red pepper
- ½ tsp. pepper and salt
- ½ pound fresh asparagus
- ½ C. chicken broth
- 1 sweet potato
- 3 minced cloves garlic
- Pepper and salt, to taste
- 1 tbsp. olive oil
- 1 pound boneless chicken breasts

How it's made:

- Cut the chicken into bite-sized chunks then eason with pepper and salt.
- Warm up the oil and add the chicken with garlic.
- Sauté the chicken for 7-10 minutes till cooked. Set the mixture to the side in a bowl.

- Using the same pan, cook the chicken broth and sweet potato for 7-10 minutes till potato is cooked and tenderized.
- Add the asparagus then cook for 4-5 minutes. Season with red pepper, pepper, and salt.

Bell Pepper Nachos

What's in it:

- 1 tbsp. red wine vinegar
- 1 tbsp. olive oil
- 2 tbsp. cilantro
- 2 tbsp. green onion
- 1 lime
- ½ C. shredded cheese
- 1 avocado
- ½ C. cherry tomatoes
- ¼ C. salsa
- 1 chopped onion
- 3 C. sliced bell peppers
- 1 pound ground beef

How it's made:

- Mix ¼ cup of onion, green onion, cilantro and cherry tomatoes together. Pour the red wine vinegar, pepper, and salt then set to the side.
- Mash the avocado with a fork. Then add ¼ cup of onion and juice of a lime then set aside.
- Warm up a tbsp of olive oil and then add the onion, sautéing till translucent in color. Pour the beef, breaking up as it cooks. Cook for 8-10 minutes then stir in the salsa. Allow to simmer 5 minutes.

- Ensure the oven is preheated to 350 degrees. On a sheet, lay out slices of bell pepper and pop into the oven for 5 minutes.
- Take the pan out and cover peppers with the meat mixture. Top with the cheese and cook for 10 minutes till cheese is melted.

Paleo Chicken Pot Pie

What's in it:

Crust:

- 6 tbsp. cold water
- 2/3 C. palm shortening
- ½ tsp. gluten-free baking powder
- 1 tsp. salt
- ½ C. tapioca flour
- 1 ½ C. blanched almond flour

Filling:

- 1/3 C. almond milk
- 1 ¾ C. chicken broth
- Pinch of paprika
- ¼ tsp. pepper
- ½ tsp. salt
- ¼ C. tapioca flour
- 1/3 C. chopped onion
- 1/3 C. butter
- 1 C. chopped broccoli
- 2 chopped carrots
- 1 pound boneless skinless chicken breasts

How it's made:

- To make the crust, mix salt, baking powder, tapioca flour, and almond flour together with a fork. Cut the shortening till mixture is similar to sand.
- Mix the cold water then put in the fridge to chill while you make the filling.
- To make the filling: Ensure the oven is preheated to 375 degrees.
- Mix the broccoli, carrots, and chicken in a pan. Cover with water. Bring to boil and boil for 10-15 minutes till chicken is cooked. Drain and set aside.
- Cook the butter and the onions together till they are tender in another pan.
- Stir in the paprika, pepper, salt, and tapioca flour in with the onions.
- Stir in the almond milk and chicken broth and simmer till thickened.
- Then remove from the heat.
- Once the dough is chilled, divide in half. Roll out ½ and place in a pie plate and put the other half back in the fridge.
- Stir the chicken mixture and butter mixtures together then pour into the crust.
- Take out the other ½ of dough. Roll it out and pour the filling.
- Put pie plate onto a baking sheet and bake for 30-35 minutes till crust is brown.
- Cool for at least 10 minutes before preparing to serve.

Bacon Wrapped Pork Tenderloin

What's in it:

6 slices sugar-free bacon
Sea salt
1/8 tsp. pepper
¼ tsp. onion powder
¼ tsp. smoked paprika
2 tbsp. brown mustard
¼ C. coconut aminos
2 tbsp. water
1/3 C. softened pitted dates
1 ½-pound pork tenderloin

How it's made:

- Cut off the silver skin and excess fat from the tenderloin. Sprinkle with the salt and put into a roasting pan.
- Ensure the oven is preheated to 400 degrees.
- Pour the dates in a blender, blending on high till a paste forms. Add the pepper, onion powder, paprika, mustard, and coconut aminos, pulsing till combined.
- Pour half of the mixture over the meat, making sure to turn over to cover.
- Put half strips of the bacon over the top of tenderloin and tuck underneath. Pour the remaining sauce over the top.
- Roast for 35-40 minutes. Then place in the broiler for 5 minutes so that the bacon turns out extra crispy. Let the meat rest for 10 minutes before cutting to serve.

Chapter 10: Paleo Dessert Recipes

Simple Reese Cups

What's in it:

- 1 C. dark chocolate chips
- 1 tbsp. honey
- 1 tbsp. coconut oil
- ½ C. unsweetened shredded coconut
- 1 C. almond butter

How it's made:

- Microwave the honey, oil and almond butter together for 30 seconds.
- Stir in the shredded coconut till combined then divide among muffin tins.
- Microwave the chocolate chips for 30 seconds till melted. Pour chocolate into the top of each tin then place in the freezer for at least 1 hour.
- Take out of the freezer.
- Using a knife, scrape around edges of cups and pop out.

Deep Dish Salted Caramel Chocolate Chip Blondies

What's in it:

Caramel:

- 1/3 C. maple syrup
- 1/3 C. almond butter
- ¼ C. melted coconut butter

Blondie:

- ¾ C. chocolate chips
- 2 tsp. vanilla extract
- 1 egg
- ¼ C. maple syrup
- ½ tsp. cinnamon
- ½ tsp. salt
- ¼ tsp. baking soda
- 1 ½ C. almond flour

How it's made:

- Ensure the oven is preheated to 350 degrees.
- Mix together the maple syrup, almond butter, and coconut oil till smooth. Then pour the mixture into a cast iron skillet.
- Combine the cinnamon, salt, baking soda, and almond flour and then add the vanilla, egg, maple, and coconut oil, stir till combined.
- Fold in the chocolate chips.
- Add to the skillet and then smooth over caramel.
- Bake for 20-25 minutes till cooked through.

Key Lime Cheesecake Bites

What's in it:

- 4 juiced and zested limes
- 3-4 tbsp. raw honey
- 1/3 C. full-fat coconut milk
- ½ C. raw cashews
- 2 tbsp. melted coconut oil
- ½ C. raw almonds

How it's made:

- With liners, line the 6 cupcake sections in a muffin tin.
- In a blender, mix coconut oil and almond together.
- Place a tbsp of the mixture into each liner to make a crust.
- Place into the freezer for 15-20 minutes.
- Puree the lime juice, honey, coconut milk, and cashews till smooth.
- Remove the tin from the freezer and fill crusts with filling. Sprinkle with lime zest and place in freezer. Chill for 4-6 hours to set.

4-Ingredient Chocolate Mousse

What's in it:

- 1/8 tsp. sea salt
- ¼ C. coconut milk
- ½ C. raw cacao powder
- 2 avocados

How it's made:

- Pour all the components into a food processor and blend till smooth.
- Pour into a sealable container and chill for 1 hour.
- Serve with a sprinkle of grated dark chocolate or coconut whipped cream. Enjoy!

Almond Joy Cookies

What's in it:

- 1-2 dashes sea salt
- 4 tbsp. raw honey
- 1 can of full-fat coconut milk
- 2/3 C. sliced almonds
- 1 C. unsweetened shredded coconut
- 1 14-ounce bag of semi-sweet mini chocolate chips

How it's made:

- To make a condensed milk, pour coconut milk into a saucepan. Pour the honey and stir.
- On low warmth, simmer for 15-25 minutes, stirring on occasion till milk thickens.
- To make cookies, ensure the oven is preheated to 325 degrees.
- Mix the condensed coconut milk, chocolate chips, almonds, and coconut together.
- Scoop out this mixture into balls using a cookie scoop.
- With a parchment paper, line a baking sheet.
- Put the almond balls onto the sheet and flatten them on top.
- Bakefor 15-20 minutes till golden.

<u>Pumpkin Coffee Cake</u>

What's in it:

- ½ tsp. salt
- ½ tsp. cinnamon
- 1 ½ tsp. pumpkin pie spice
- ½ tsp. baking soda
- ¼ C. coconut flour
- 4 eggs
- 1 C. canned pumpkin
- ¼ C. coconut sugar
- ¼ C. maple syrup
- ¼ C. melted coconut oil

Crumb Topping:

- 2 tbsp. coconut oil
- 2 tbsp. maple syrup
- ½ tsp. cinnamon
- 2 tbsp. coconut sugar
- ½ C. almond flour
- ¼ C. coconut flour

How it's made:

- Ensure the oven is preheated to 325 degrees. With a parchment paper, line a 9x9 baking dish.
- Combine all of the crumb topping components together till it resembles a wet sand.
- Then combine the pumpkin, coconut sugar, maple syrup, and coconut oil.
- Whisk together the eggs and then add to mixture.
- Then add the remaining dry ingredients, combining well. Ensure that there are no dry pockets within mixture before pouring into the pan.
- Top with crumb topping then bake for 45-50 minutes.

Paleo Sex in a Pan

What's in it:

Crust:
- 4 tbsp. coconut oil
- ¾ C. dates
- 1 ½ C. pecans

Second Layer:

- 1 pinch salt
- 2 tsp. apple cider vinegar
- 1/3 C. shortening
- 2/3 C. cashew butter

Third Layer:

- 1 tsp. vanilla extract
- 2 tbsp. honey
- ½ C. coconut milk
- ¼ C. coconut flour
- 1/3 C. arrowroot flour

Fourth Layer:

- 2 tbsp. honey
- ½ C. cocoa powder
- ½ C. shortening
- ½ C. coconut milk

Fifth Layer:

- 4 tbsp. honey
- 1 ½ C. shortening

Sixth Layer:

- Grated 80%+ cacao dark chocolate

How it's made:

- Roughly chop the pecans and then place the pecans and dates into a food processor. Grind till crumbly. Stir in the coconut oil and then press mixture into the bottom of a cake pan.
- Put in the fridge to chill.
- Combine all of the 2nd layer components and pour over the chilled crust then chill.
- Mix together all of the 3rd layer components and pour over the 2nd layer then chill.
- Combine all of the 4th layer components and pour over the 3rd layer then chill.
- Mix all of the 5th later components and pour over the 4th layer then chill.
- Grate the chocolate directly over the entire dish. Chill for at least ½ an hour. Then slice into pieces and serve!

Fudgy Avocado Brownies

What's in it:

- ½ C. coconut flour
- ½ C. cocoa powder
- 3 eggs
- 1 tsp. vanilla
- ½ C. honey
- 2 avocados
- 2 tbsp. coconut oil
- 300g dark chocolate

Avocado Frosting:

- 3 tbsp. maple syrup
- 3 tbsp. unsweetened cocoa powder
- 1 avocado

How it's made:

- Ensure the oven is preheated to 400 degrees. With a parchment paper, line a 9x13 dish.
- In a glass bowl, melt the coconut oil and chocolate together over simmering water till smooth.
- Put the avocado in a processor and blend till smooth.
- Stir together the vanilla, avocado, and honey into cooled chocolate. Then add the eggs, one at a time.
- Add the coconut flour and cocoa powder, stirring till batter becomes smooth.
- Pour batter into pan and smooth the top then bake for 12-15 minutes.
- To make the frosting, pour all the components into a food processor then blend till smooth. Spread over cooled brownies. Cut into 24 pieces.

Double Chocolate Cookies

What's in it:

- 1 C. semi-sweet chocolate chips
- 1 egg
- 1 ½ tsp. vanilla
- 6 tbsp. natural almond butter
- ¾ C. coconut sugar
- 7 tbsp. coconut oil

- ¼ tsp. salt
- 1 tsp. baking soda
- 1/3 C. + 4 tsp. cocoa powder
- ¼ C. coconut flour
- ¾ C. almond flour

How it's made:

- Stir the salt, baking soda, cocoa powder, coconut flour, and almond flour together.
- Beat the fat and sugar on medium speed till combined. Then beat the flour and vanilla, then the egg. Stir your flour mixture, combining thoroughly.
- Ensure the oven is preheated to 350 degrees. With a parchment paper, line a baking sheet.
- Roll the dough into balls and roll in the remaining chocolate chips. Place 3" apart onto the sheet.
- Bake for 11-14 minutes till the center no longer looks wet. Cookies will be soft.
- Allow to cool completely before serving.

Conclusion

Thank you for reading *Paleo Diet – Don't Harm Yourself.*

I hope that the contents of this book find you motivated to begin incorporating the Paleo lifestyle into your very own life! I hope that you were able to get the tools you need to achieve your goals of becoming a healthier version of yourself through the tips, tricks, and valuable information that you just absorbed.

The next step is to put your newly acquired knowledge to the test in your very own life. Each diet offers various results for different people, but unless you take the first step into implementing it into your everyday lifestyle, you will never come to find out what it can do for you!

You don't have to live like a caveman but I hope you will be able to see the amazing benefits from eating like one as you begin your trek into the Paleo Diet. Good luck!

Finally, If you enjoyed this book and you thought it was a solid and informative read, I'd love to see your review on Amazon. Your opinion can really help somebody to benefit from this book as well

(To leave a honest review on amazon, please scan the QR code below through your mobile device or tablet)

(Or simply go to the link below on your web browser)

https://goo.gl/oLCvjL

Thank you!

**Great! You've Made It To The End!
As I Promised, Here Is Your FREE BONUS Of 4
Valuable Reports For Weight Loss And Healthy Eating
(Value $27).**

To download a free bonus please scan the QR code below to your mobile device or tablet.

Or Simply Use This Link:

https://annetteloveblog.lpages.co/paleo-diet-free-bonus-1/

Check Out My Other Books

Below you'll find some of my other books that are popular on Amazon and Kindle as well. Simply scan QR code below to check it out. Alternatively, you can visit my author page on Amazon to see other work done by me.

<u>- Keto Diet, Don't Harm Yourself: How To Avoid TOP 5 Mistakes on Ketogenic Diet. Keto Guide For Beginners, Includes Meal Plan For Weight Loss, Cookbook and Recipes, Body Healing Plan, Improving Metabolism and Nutrition Facts + Bonus Chapters</u>

If the QR code does not work, for whatever reason, you can simply search for these titles on the Amazon website to find them by typing in amazon's search bar – *keto diet don't harm yourself* or *keto meal plan*

Preview Of 'Keto Diet – Don't Harm Yourself'

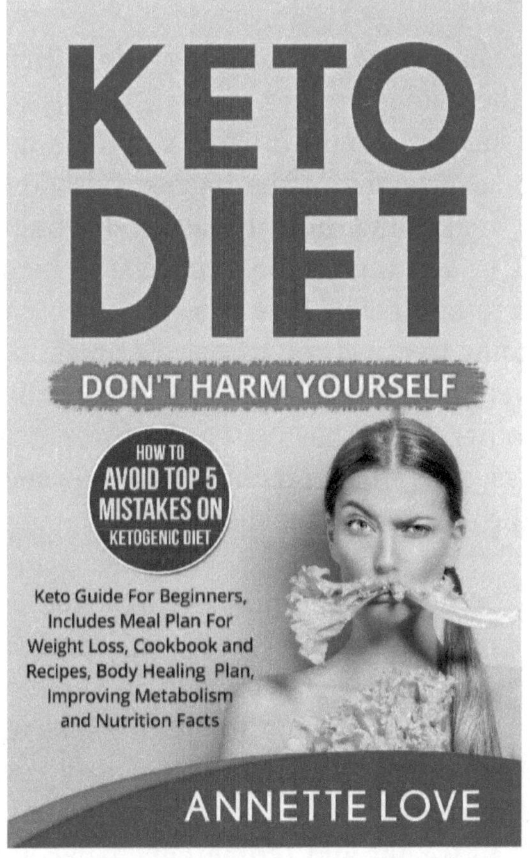

Introduction

Congratulations on downloading *Keto Diet, Don't Harm Yourself* and thank you for doing so.

The following chapters will discuss everything that you need to know about the ketogenic diet, as well as steps that you can take to avoid harming yourself while you're on it. This book is also going to cover some of the biggest mistakes that people new to keto make and how to avoid making those same mistakes. We'll talk about the *realities* of keto. Everybody always wants to talk about how keto is some savior of a meal plan that is going to cause you to lose a tremendous amount of weight with very little work. While this is partially true, keto is just like any other diet. It has its set of problems that you'll run into as well as a set of "best practices" that you should follow in order to get the most out of the diet.

Now, there is a slight separation between the ketogenic diet and other diets. While other diets can very much be considered "fads", the ketogenic diet is grounded in very sound science. It's been used for a long time for both rapid weight loss in morbidly obese patients as well as to control severe seizures. It's a medically safe diet and the science behind it can make you lose a lot of weight and ultimately change your life. We'll go more into that in the first chapter.

However, it is not a miracle diet. It's going to take work and careful attention and, like any other major lifestyle change, you're going to have to be extremely careful about what you're putting in your body.

Chapter 1: Keto for Beginners (and Possible Consequences)

So you've made it this far and by now you're probably wondering what exactly keto *is*. After all, there are mentions of the diet pretty much everywhere. Even celebrities have started to espouse the numerous virtues of the ketogenic diet.

LeBron James turned to a ketogenic version of the Paleo diet in order to lose some weight; Gwyneth Paltrow is releasing a low-carb cookbook called *It's All Good!* and tries to avoid giving her kids carbohydrates, and even Kim Kardashian used a low-carb diet similar to keto in order to shed around sixty pounds of baby weight. So what are they all trying to get at, here?

The ketogenic diet is pretty easy to understand at its core. The thing that makes it different from Paleo is that Paleo's focus is on eating solely unprocessed food, but Paleo permits natural sugars like honey and high-sugar fruits. Meanwhile, keto focuses on restricting carbs. The thing which sets Keto apart from Atkins is that Atkins *starts off* with a ketogenic diet (called the induction phase) which then morphs into something else, adding back in carbs and aiming for a "sustainable" diet.

Keto is based on some essential scientific components that can be a little dense though. Let's start at the beginning.

First off, as you may or may not know, there are three primary components to food known as *macronutrients*. These are *fat, protein,* and *carbohydrates,* and all of them are important in their own way in the context of the body's function. For example, fat lubricates the bloodstream and reinforces cell structure. Protein provides essential muscle structure and keeps you strong. Carbohydrates serve the primary function of giving the body energy and spurring essential operations.

The ketogenic diet is based on the idea of *ketones....*

https://www.amazon.com/Keto-Diet-Dont-Harm-Yourself-ebook/dp/B074XF4B6R

What Other People Say About Keto Diet – Don't Harm Yourself

⭐⭐⭐⭐⭐ **I like this book.**

By Landon Hayden on September 21, 2017

Format: Kindle Edition | Verified Purchase

This book is ideal for those that attempting try are attempting to slim within the right manner while not harming their body and you'll learn some sensible and healthy recipes that you just will try reception. This book is incredibly well written by the author and that i suggest this book to all.

⭐⭐⭐⭐⭐ **I definately learned lots of new things about the diet.**

By Rock on September 20, 2017

Format: Kindle Edition | Verified Purchase

Fantastic book that merges both the personal and scientific aspects of a low carb, high fat diet. I devoured this book very quickly as it was just a pleasure to read. I bought the kindle version, but I'm probably going to get a paper back copy too.

⭐⭐⭐⭐⭐ **This is a great book, since I have been hearing a lot ...**

By Jessica on September 4, 2017

Format: Kindle Edition | Verified Purchase

This is a great book, since I have been hearing a lot about the Keto diet,I finally decided to take a closer look at what it really is. I was so impressed. This book has great recipes to follow, I already tried 5 and the food was delicious.

⭐⭐⭐⭐⭐ **This Book is a Gem! Thanks**

By Beatrice on September 21, 2017

Format: Kindle Edition | Verified Purchase

I have been doing keto for a year know. I've read a ton of information about keto and listen to keto postcard as well. This book is incredibly well written by the author and that i suggest this book. Her whole foods approach to keto is refreshing. This is a beautiful tome of a book, well researched and well written.

https://www.amazon.com/Keto-Diet-Dont-Harm-Yourself-ebook/dp/B074XF4B6R

Or go to: http://amzn.to/2hpfzQI

Appendix 1: Conversion table

I understand that it might get confusing with measurements when trying to cook something delicious, so for your convenience I've decided to include the Conversion table. I hope this will help you to dive deeper into tasty Keto recipes that are provided in this book. Enjoy!

Oven Temperature Conversions

Fahrenheit	Celsius	Gas Mark
250 F	130 C	1/2
275 F	140 C	1
300 F	150 C	2
325 F	165 C	3
350 F	177 C	4
375 F	190 C	5
400 F	200 C	6
425 F	220 C	7
450 F	230 C	8
475 F	245 C	9
500 F	260 C	10

Liquid Volumes

Imperial (UK)	Metric	U.S.
½ fl oz	15 ml	1 tbsp
1 fl oz	30 ml	1/8 cup
2 fl oz	55 ml	¼ cup
3 fl oz	85 ml	1/3 cup
4 fl oz	115 ml	½ cup
5 fl oz	140 ml	2/ cup
6 fl oz	170 ml	¾ cup
7 fl oz	200 ml	7/8 cup
8 fl oz	230 ml	1 cup
16 fl oz	455 ml	2 cups (1 US pint)
20 fl oz (1 UK pint)	570 ml	2 ½ cups

Weights

Metric	Imperial
15 g	1/ oz
30 g	1 oz
60 g	2 oz
90 g	3 oz
125 g	4 oz
175 g	6 oz
250 g	8 oz
300 g	10 oz
375 g	12 oz
400 g	13 oz
425 g	14 oz
500 g	1 lb
750 g	1 ½ lb
1 kg	2 lb